Laughing My Butt Off

How I Lost Over 125 Pounds Without Pills, Surgery, or Alfalfa Sprouts

John W. Turner

DEDICATION

To Abby, my granddaughter.

All this is for you. I want to be alive
to see you grow up.

CONTENTS

ACKNOWLEDGMENTS

A multitude of thanks to   Linda, Jennifer, Melissa, and Sarah. All of you have made this a reality.

A huge thanks goes out to my wife, Gloria. You have stuck with me through all my varying sizes. I'm so very glad that I didn't roll over and crush you. I love you!

Thank you to Julie for editing this book.

Thanks to R.A. Higbee for the cover photography.

Medical Disclaimer: This book is for educational and informational purposes only and may not be construed as medical advice. The information is not intended to replace medical advice offered by physicians.

INTRODUCTION

I am a comedian, pastor, poet, author, encourager, spiritual advisor, husband, stepfather, grandfather, brother, uncle, cousin, and a myriad of other titles. My least favorite designation is "fat."

A couple years ago, I registered 324 pounds at the doctor's office. I know I weighed more before that visit. I would not be surprised to know I had been 350 pounds.

I hated being fat. Truthfully, I really hated myself. I tried so many things to lose the weight, only to lose a little and then gain it all back, plus some.

Everything changed in January of 2016.

This book is a brief look at how it felt for me to be overweight, how I have lost over 125 pounds, and how you can do the same.

Purposely, this book is not lengthy. I don't want you to spend weeks reading a book. I want you to begin losing the weight that you want to lose.

I have inserted some of my jokes throughout this book. There is no rhyme nor reason as to where they are located. I want you to laugh. Morbid obesity, diabetes, the weight struggle, self esteem issues, etc., are not laughing matters. But, my sense of humor kept the pain of my condition from getting the best of me.

My new book will be coming out soon. It's called "1001 Ways To Help Your Overweight Friend." Here's point one: Shut up and buy him a pizza.

I hope this book helps you.

1 ZIPPED OR UNZIPPED?

An honor turned into a horror in about fifteen seconds.

I was asked to be the keynote speaker at the graduation service of a small college. I was thrilled to no end to have been given such a wonderful privilege. Prior to the event, I called Robert, the event coordinator, to find out the attire for the evening. He told me that there was no need to wear a suit or coat, just wear a nice white shirt, because I would be given a graduation gown to wear.

I envy people that can put their cell phone in their back pocket. Once I get "me" into my jeans, there's no room for anything else.

When I arrived at the ceremony, Robert handed me a gown to put on. It didn't fit. I asked if there was a larger size. There wasn't. Robert said, "Just wear it with the zipper down." It zipped from the front. Then I heard these words: "Lots of people wear them unzipped."

My wife said, "I like a man with meat on his bones." So, I gained 100 pounds. Then she says, "I like a little meat, not the whole meat market."

Reluctantly, I put the robe on, left the zipper down, and made my way to a mirror. Wearing a black gown, with my bright white shirt exposed, made me look like the world's largest Oreo cookie. I wanted to crawl in a hole. But I couldn't, I was the keynote speaker. I was there to bring a word of congratulations and challenge to these young men and women who were stepping out into new ventures.

> *Y'all ever seen that TV show "Sit and Get Fit?" Well... I sat and got fat.*

I can't get those words out of my head: "Lots of people wear them unzipped." I haven't seen all those people. In fact, I have seen only one of them: me.

I hated myself that evening for being so big that I couldn't wear the graduation robe.

After all the embarrassment, I went home and ate two packages of Oreos. They have never embarrassed me.

2 FREEDOM OR FRITOS?

Growing up, meals at home were pretty predictable. Most dinners consisted of a hamburger patty or meatloaf, a vegetable or two, a slice of bread, macaroni and cheese or mash potatoes, and some kind of a dessert. And that was it. By "that" I mean, there was not a going back for seconds or thirds. What was put on our plate was all there was. Period.

Then… the sweet taste of freedom. Going off to college.

> *I went to McDonald's for breakfast. The attendant asked me the silliest question: "Do you want a pie with that?" Of course, I do.*

I was making my own money, paying my own way, and this freedom spilled over into my eating habits. No longer was I limited to what my parents provided and put on my plate. I ate what I wanted, when I wanted, and how much I wanted. It was tacos, burritos, Oreos, Doritos, French fries, etc.

> *My doctor took me off cheese. I wonder if she realizes that means she also took me off broccoli and cauliflower.*

John W. Turner

You name it, I ate it, and lots of it. I thought I was free. I wasn't. This unhealthy lifestyle put me on the fast train to morbid obesity.

3 TABLE OR BOOTH?

As much fun as the restaurant experience is supposed to be, when you are overweight, it can be a disaster. The horror begins in the lobby. The hostess asks, "Table or booth?" As always, the answer is "Table."

Since most people hate their jobs and most people love pizza, shouldn't most people work for Pizza Hut?

On this particular occasion, I added, "The booths are always too small for me."

After I eat, it looks like a crime scene.

The hostess said, "Ours are a lot bigger. You won't have any trouble fitting in."

She led my wife and me to our booth, placed the menus on the table, and just left before I had a chance to sit. Easily, my wife seated herself.

They tell me to substitute cauliflower for potatoes. What's next? Instead of chocolate chips, rabbit droppings?

Then the circus began. I did my

best contortionist act to try to get in.
Fail. I tried to suck my gut in. Fail.
I then tried to position the table
between my ripples of fat. Fail.
There was no way I was getting in.

> *My weight loss knowledge has spiritual roots. I learned most of it from Nun of the Above.*

So I stood beside our table, doing
the Stand of Shame, for what
seemed like an eternity, to get the
hostess' attention. I felt like a fool
standing there. Finally she reseated
us at a table.

> *Congratulate me on my lifestyle changes. This week I only gained 5 pounds.*

As horrible as I felt, I didn't let

that feeling keep me from enjoying some quite delicious buttered breadsticks.

4 CHAIRS AND CHEEKS

For most people, family get togethers are a lot of fun. They weren't fun for me when I was overweight.

> *I do a new exercise called "Push Downs." It's basically just keeping myself in bed.*

On one particular occasion, before I was married, my future in-laws invited me to join the family for a cook out. As soon as I arrived, I could see there was going to be trouble. Small lawn chairs.

I told me wife, "Honey, I will always stick with you. Seriously... as big as I am, I can't run."

I was pointed in the direction of a wooden chair. Poor chair. It never had a chance. I tried pretending to sit, by not putting all of my weight on the chair. I held that position for about four or five seconds. Then I ran out of strength and was forced to let all of me rest on the chair. I could feel it beginning to buckle. I could also hear it cracking. But before I could get up, that poor chair gave up the ghost, and deposited my big self on the lawn.

> *A lady tried to impress me on my healthy walk today by carrying two 5 pound dumbbells. I said, "That's nothing, lady. I'm carrying an extra 80 pounds."*

Different family members immediately rushed to me. "Can we help you up? Can we help you up?" I said, "No. But you can help me get the wooden splinters out of my butt crack." It was embarrassing to say the least.

The barbecue, however, was delicious. And more important than that, there was lots of it.

5 MOONLIGHT OR MOONPIES?

I didn't want to be overweight.

After I gained the first 30 pounds of extra weight, I started thinking about how to get it off.

> *I'm totally exhausted from my workout at the YMCA and all I did was the song.*

I was in college. A few of my friends knew I was interested in knocking off the weight, so they encouraged me to go walking with them. I let them know that I wasn't that fast and would probably have a hard time keeping up with them. They said, "Don't worry. We just walk casually. You won't have a problem sticking with us."

> *I have a new fitness coach that's doing wonders for me. He's exactly what I need. Focused, experienced, and former military. His name is Colonel Sanders.*

Most evenings, at about 10:30, they would leave the dorm and walk for an hour or so.

So I went with them. Reluctantly.

The college was situated on a hill and the surrounding community had several little hills. We all started walking, talking, and having a great time. Actually, it was killing me, but I never said a word.

You know when you don't get all your items at the drive-thru, is that called an "eating disorder?"

Up and down hill one. No problem. Hill two. A breeze. Hill three. Success. Then, all of a sudden, my friends started jogging. I jogged three steps and hit my limit.

A friend of mine ended a relationship and as a result gained about 120 pounds. He broke up with Jenny Craig.

I hollered, "Hey guys! I thought we were going to walk?!" My voice echoed down the hill at about the same pace they were jogging.

No one heard me.

> *They say that getting out of bed is half the battle. I sure hope so because I'm getting back into the bed to finish the battle.*

I thought for sure they would stop at the bottom of the hill and wait for me. They didn't.

I watched them reach the end of the block at the bottom of the hill.

> *My favorite fantasy movie is "Lord of the Onion Rings."*

Then they began to run.

I took a few more steps and sat down on the curb.

> *When losing weight, people have said, "I can see it in your face." What does that even mean? From the neck down am I still a big fat tub of lard?*

I sat there for a few minutes.

I was very upset.

The people that I thought were my support group turned out to be the farthest thing from it.

I was angry. First at me. Then at them.

If I just wasn't so fat this would

never have happened.

I sat on the curb for about 20 minutes. Alone, except for my thoughts.

The family asked me to be the anchor for the Balloon Bouncy Castle. See... not everyone is supposed to lose weight.

It was a beautiful night, except for what I had just experienced. The moon shone brightly that night and as her beams shined on me like a spotlight, all I could think of was how I could sure use a moonpie about now.

6 REAL OR FAKE?

My weight has been a wrestling match. So I guess it was no surprise the day that I crossed paths with professional wrestler, Jimmy Wehba, also known as Skandor Akbar. God bless his memory.

> *I'm in a 12 step fitness program. It's 12 steps from the recliner to the refrigerator.*

When I met Mr. Wehba, he was

working with the Global Wrestling Federation and using the name "The Godfather of Wrestling." This was in the 1980's.

At the time, Mr. Wehba was involved with a company that sold nutritional items. A friend of mine suggested that I buy a healthy tea that would aid in my weight loss. I bought several boxes. It tasted horrible. But I was faithful to drinking it for several weeks. It did absolutely nothing for me other than make me want to eat and drink things that I shouldn't just to get the horrible taste out of my mouth.

They say, "Go big or go home." Obviously, I didn't go home.

Even though professional

wrestling is not real, my struggle with my weight was very real. I was in the midst of trying anything that would help me lose my extra 50 pounds. It was as if opponent after opponent stepped in the ring and each one pinned me to the mat keeping me from losing weight.

> *I needed change in my life. So, I swallowed a roll of quarters.*

I like watching professional wrestling even with knowing that it is fake. I realize that it is a complete waste of my time. I have found the same to be true of all the weight loss teas, tablets, and bars.

Would I ever find a way to win against weight? Or, would I be forever destined to stay in the wrestling ring?

It was no fun being overweight.

Being pinned to the mat by obesity was no way to live.

> *I saw a professional wrestler throw out the first pitch of a baseball game. See? I always knew baseball was fake.*

Professional wrestling may be fake, but the battle against weight is very real.

7 BIG AND BIGGER

In my early days as a pastor, I was introduced to George, a preacher that lived across the country. I was told that he could help me and the church that I was pastoring.

Definition of "bench press:" making myself stay seated at the picnic table while eating 27 hotdogs.

George and I talked regularly on the phone. He gave me some great insights that were extremely helpful in the ministry. He told me that he was coming to Texas and would love to speak to our church. So I scheduled George for a 3 day conference.

In my fitness journey, I get a lot of assistance from Hamburger Helper.

The day George arrived, he met me at the church. I was straightening some things up on the platform when George entered the sanctuary. I was given ample warning that he was about to enter the room. The light from the sun that was shining through the entry door was completely blocked by George's body. He was huge, and I don't mean tall.

As he walked down the aisle to meet me, I was feeling like the little shepherd boy David being approached by Goliath.

> *You know the best way to help a hamburger? With cheese... and three more hamburgers on the side.*

At the time, I was weighing about 250, 60 or 70 pounds over what I should have weighed. George must have been over 400 pounds.

As we met in the aisle of the church, I could tell that George noticed my girth. The first words out of his mouth to me were: "We're going to get along just fine together this weekend!"

Up to that point, I didn't see my

weight as that "big" of a concern. I knew I was a little overweight, but never in my wildest dreams did I associate myself as being in the same category as this preacher that I just met.

> *Two words from your doctor can change everything. Like: "Weight's down." "Cholesterol's good." And of course, "Bend over."*

But George was right. We did get along fine that weekend. When we were not in the middle of a church service, we were at a restaurant eating. Since his visits to Texas were rare, he had to get caught up on Texas cuisine... and lots of it. Sadly, I didn't mind being his partner in crime.

That weekend of services was just the beginning of many trips that my new preacher friend George made to Texas. Every time he visited, we hit all his favorite eating spots. Sometimes it was Mexican food. Other times, barbecue. Occasionally, burgers.

When it comes to getting healthy, truthfully, I'm looking for more of a 1.2 step program.

At one barbecue restaurant, George could never get full on one plate, even if was the double meat plate. But that wasn't going to be a problem for George. He would go to the condiment bar, grab a couple of rolls, tear them open, and fill them with onion and pickle slices. He called them "onion sandwiches."

After a few of those, his hunger was satiated.

It was weird the first time I experienced George eating onion sandwiches. But the weird would soon wear away because it would not be long until I would be the one eating onion sandwiches after eating a large plate of barbecue.

My weight gain was caused by bees: burgers, burritos, and buttered biscuits.

Fast forward a few years. George got concerned about his weight. He even dropped a few pounds. But his schedule of preaching on the road, kept George from making any serious headway in his desire to lose weight. Whatever pounds were lost when he was at home, would soon be found when he spent weekends preaching at churches like mine.

Shortly before George's next trip to Texas, I got word from his wife that he died from a massive heart attack.

I don't understand why I can't have donuts. How could something shaped like a halo be bad for me?

I should have heeded the handwriting on the wall. The message was loud and clear. I was going to be next. But I refused to obey it. I was too busy eating onion sandwiches.

8 JOHN OR BIG JOHN

Dale Carnegie, one of the founders of the self-help and motivation movement, said, "A person's name is to that person, the sweetest, most important sound in any language." If that's true, and I personally believe it is, something ugly happens inside a person when his or her name is distorted.

Once I became obviously overweight, people began to call me

"Big John." I hated that and I still do. Some had the audacity to tell me that it was a term of endearment. Some said that they called me "Big John" because of the country and western song with the same name. I, for one, do not for one second believe that. I felt that people called me "Big John" because of my weight, not my height.

I shop at the Big and Tall store because I'm tall, of course.

I have had people that just met me begin calling me "Big John."

I have always been too kind to say anything about this until now.

If I wasn't already having a bad day, someone calling me "Big John" would make certain I had a bad day.

> *I recently read that small changes can lead to big weight loss. So I made some small changes. I went from eating 3 meals to four, 1 burger to two, and from little exercise to none.*

I will never forget the evening when I was working in the grocery store. I was an assistant service manager and my duties took me all over the store. When I was at the farthest point at the back of the store, I was called to the front to handle a customer complaint. The person at the customer service desk got on the intercom and announced to the whole store, "Big John, please come to customer service. Big John to customer service."

I was livid. To me, this was degrading, insulting, and very disrespectful. It pains me to this day to even recall this incident.

I just wanted to crawl in a hole. I had been called "Big John" more times than I could count. But this was the first time that I was called by that name over an intercom.

My favorite science fiction movie is "E.T.: Extra Tortillas."

The woman who did this could tell by the look on my face that she had done the wrong thing. Thankfully, she never did it again. Honestly, I don't know what I would have done if she had given a repeat performance.

To some people, the overweight are treated like we have been put on the planet just so people can make fun of us.

Most of us, like myself, just grin and bear it. We just receive those painful words and hide them on the inside.

I was told that to lose weight I should eat more small meals. So I eat a small breakfast at 6:00, another one at 6:15, an additional breakfast at 6:30, one more at 6:45...

When I was packing on the extra pounds, I knew I was overweight. It was no surprise. All the X's on the label of my shirts and the size 50 on my pants were constant reminders. The very last thing I needed was an audible reminder from someone calling me "Big John."

As a pastor, people have called me a lot of different things: Brother, Pastor, Minister, Reverend, etc. I encourage people to call me "John." That was the name my parents gave me when I entered into this world. I love my name.

My family and those who knew me when I was a kid, usually call me "Johnny." That's okay… for them only. For everyone else, I'm John.

Obesity is in my genes, and also in my shirts, and socks.

I am not Big John.

Not now. Not then. Not ever.

9 JUDGE AND JURY

I went to court and it was one of the most humiliating experiences of my life. It was the Supreme Court.

Years ago, there was a chain of fitness clubs that had racquetball courts and they were called Supreme Courts.

I'm from a big family. There's not that many of us, but we're huge.

I had not been a pastor for very long and church members were already concerned about my size. Jess, one of our church members, talked to me almost every Sunday after the service about how beneficial it was to go to the gym every day. I really didn't want to hear it. I just wanted to go eat.

Weight loss is magic. It's not pulling a rabbit out of a hat; it's pulling your hand out of the chip bag.

For Christmas, Jess and his family gave me the worst gift ever: a membership to Supreme Court. This put me in a quandary. I didn't want to go and I didn't want to upset a family in the church.

Maybe it was just in my mind, but

I was led to believe that Jess and I would be working out together.

I will never forget the first time I showed up at the gym. I was wearing shorts and a sweat shirt. And I never, ever, wore shorts. Not for anything.

After getting rained on during my walk at lunch, one of my co-workers said, "You look like you've been in a wet tee-shirt contest." I said, "Don't laugh. I won."

As I walked in, all I saw were people who did not need to be working out. I felt totally out of place.

I looked for Jess, but he was nowhere to be found.

No one on staff offered any assistance.

I walked from machine to machine trying to figure out what they did and what I was supposed to do. It seemed as if I was in a torture chamber and these were the instruments of pain.

All eyes were on the big guy. Or, that was what I thought.

My struggle with sweets is working to my advantage. I've been cast to star in a movie. A horror movie. "Children of the Candy Corn."

I could hear what they were thinking. "I hope he doesn't break that machine." "How much does he weigh?" "What a slob."

I was in Hell.

It was the worst hour of my life.

After wandering around the gym, I left.

> *An image of a tortilla appeared on my painting of The Virgin Mary.*

A few weeks went by and Jess realized I wasn't going to the gym. He asked why. I told him. But that wasn't enough for Jess. He had to let me know that his very expensive gift had been a waste.

Thanks Jess.

That encounter let me feel terrible about the gym from a completely different angle.

> *I called an exorcist to get the Fat Demon out. After an hour of praying over me, he said, "It's not a demon. It's all you."*

People who have never struggled with their weight, in my opinion, have no idea of what it's like to be in an overweight person's shoes. If they could spend a week in Fatville, maybe they would be a little more understanding.

I never went back to the Supreme Court.

I drove away as fast as I could to the nearest Taco Bell and had a great meal that started off with a Burrito Supreme.

Laughing My Butt Off

Thank you Taco Bell. You have never made me feel embarrassed to walk through your doors.

10 WARNING SIGNS OR DINNER BELLS?

Back in the late 1980's and early 1990's, I spent every Saturday morning conducting a church service at the local nursing home.

> *I used to believe that "the only thing to fear is fear itself" until my doctor put me on a diet.*

It was one of the highlights of my

week… for the most part.

The residents who attended the service seemed to really appreciate it. Some of the church members would go with me. Usually there was live music. Some of the residents who did not have all their mental faculties would hear the music and think it was a dance. And they would dance. They enjoyed their dancing, even if it was to "Amazing Grace" and "What a Friend We Have in Jesus."

> *When our house was broken into, I was devastated… until I saw they stole our treadmill.*

After the service, the attendees were always appreciative and very complimentary. At least most of them were.

Some of them told me exactly what was on their mind. About once a month, I would get a lecture about my weight. I'd hear their stories of all the fat people they knew that died prematurely. As they gave me their unsolicited counsel to lose weight, it only made me push their wheelchair a little faster to their room.

> *I lost 60 pounds just by going to the mall. If anyone sees my nephew, please call me.*

I was there to preach to them, not have them preach to me.

One particular Saturday, none of

my helpers showed up. It was going to be a solo act. The staff had not put out any chairs for the mobile residents. So, the job of carrying chairs from one end of the facility to the other, became mine that day.

After I carried the second load of chairs, I began to feel weak. I was out of breath and thought I was going to pass out. I leaned against a stack of chairs to catch my breath. Thankfully, after a minute or two, I recovered. Had any of the staff seen me, they might have admitted me to the nursing home that day.

Studies reveal that exposure to cold temperatures prompt weight loss. So... the slurpee, snow cone, and Klondike bar diet begins today.

This was a warning. A wakeup call. An attention getter. But like the previous ones, this one too was ignored.

> *I'm so out of shape that when I go for a walk, I don't sunburn... I slow roast.*

Why did I not heed the warnings? I don't even know. But I do know, regrettably, I always heeded my hunger pangs.

After the service that day, instead of making any changes to my lifestyle, I just changed my order at Wendy's and added another cheeseburger.

11 EXCESS AND ELASTIC

To me it's absolutely mind blowing how some people feel they have the liberty to say whatever they want to someone that is overweight. No restraint. No forethought. Just any and everything goes.

After many trips to WalMart being disappointed that they didn't have my size in pants, I decided to go to a store that specialized in men's clothes. I walked in and noticed they had a "Big and Tall" department, so I headed over there.

> *One lady at church used to judge me and say, "You're fat. Gluttony is a sin." Every Sunday, she'd say, "Overeating is wrong." Then one Sunday she told me, "The way you eat is sinful. You need to read John 3:16." I said, "Lady, read John 3:16? I am John 3:16!"*

A clerk, a very friendly young man, followed me and asked if he could help me. I told him what I wanted and he measured my waist and inseam. He found a pair of black slacks that were my size.

He said, "You should get a pair of Oops pants."

I responded, "What are Oops pants."

"They are pants that have an elastic waste band that stretch one or two extra inches for when you gain."

> *My favorite western movie is "A Fistful of Doritos."*

Sounded innocent enough, to him. He was just trying to be helpful. But when those words fell on my ears, they sounded a whole lot like: "I can tell that you are certainly not on the way to losing weight, you big fat slob." And this man didn't even know me.

What I really needed was a pair of Super Oops pants that would stretch a foot or two. But I certainly wasn't going to admit that to this young man.

I walked out that day with my first of many Oops pants.

I was told to write down everything I eat. Keep a food journal. The more I wrote the hungrier I got.

The only redeeming element to that encounter was that there was a Burger King nearby. They never make me feel bad. They always treat me like royalty, just like a king.

12 HEALTH BARS AND HEMORRHOIDS

Shopping is a nightmare when you are obese.

If you have ever shopped at WalMart for clothes, you know that they have their jeans on shelves. Usually they are all mixed up. But if you should happen to be lucky and find them organized, you will discover that they placed the smaller sizes on top and the larger sizes on the bottom.

So shopping for jeans at WalMart always meant that I would be on my hands and knees sorting through the bottom shelf for jeans my size, that usually were not there. I always felt like they had a camera on me. "Let's film the fat guy bending over, stooping down, trying to get up... so we can have something to submit to America's Funniest Home Videos."

> *I wrote down every single thing I ate for 24 months. Guess what happened? I got Carpal Tunnel Syndrome.*

But it was far from funny.

And then there's the pricing. Why

is it that jeans in size 32, 34, 36, 38 are all the same price, but add 2 inches and you pay 2 to 4 dollars more? What is it about those two inches that are more expensive?

Have you ever been to Casual Male? It's a big and tall men's clothing store where, to me, they casually charge $80 to $100 for a shirt that you could get at WalMart for $12 if they carried size 4X.

Writing down everything I eat has really helped me.... become a great speller.

As bad as shopping for clothes is, grocery shopping is even worse.

When you are overweight, you feel as if everyone is looking at what you put in your grocery cart. I can hear their thoughts. "He doesn't need Doritos." "He's probably never been in the produce department." "Look. He thinks the Diet Cokes are going to undo the damage."

Before food journaling, I couldn't spell "fried zucchini with artichoke dip."

Even worse is going through the checkout. I never had a checker say anything about my selection, but I sure felt like I was being judged. It was so bad that I would buy distraction items. I'd buy 16 glue boards to catch mice or 7 tubes of Preparation H just to give the checker something to think about other than what I was going to be eating.

You would think it would be better when I was buying health bars or meal replacement shakes. It wasn't. It felt like I was just calling attention to the fact that I was overweight.

No matter how you try to trick me, "healthy lifestyle plan" still sounds a whole lot like a diet.

The weekly trip to the store became one of my many never-ending nightmares.

13 LIES AND FRIES

It has been said that "You can run, but you can't hide." I wish that was true, because I can't run either.

For a long time I lived a lie concerning my weight.

Whenever I would be invited to go eat with friends or go to someone's house for a meal, I would always eat a lot less than I actually wanted to. I would be offered more, and would say, "Oh. No thanks. I'm full." Or, "I'm cutting back." And then someone would compliment me on working on my weight.

My wife calls me her "hot salsa." I thought it was a compliment until I read the bottle, which says: "thick and chunky."

It was just a façade. As soon as the event was over, I would make a mad dash to the nearest fast food establishment and load up.

Whenever I went to my doctor, once again, I would be lying through my teeth.

One of my lies began a couple of days before my appointment. I would have gone almost 3 months without doing anything that my doctor had told me to do. So, three or four days before I would see my doctor, I would walk a few blocks, try cutting back, skip a meal or two. I would do anything to make the scales show at least one pound of weight loss. That way I could tell my doctor that I had been working on my weight.

Chewing sugar-free gum helps you conquer cravings. Chewing on 16 tacos works even better.

It was a lie. And it didn't work. My doctor ended up doing the same thing every time: increasing the dosage of a pill she had already prescribed or add another one to my list.

After every visit to the doctor, after getting the bad news that I always received, after promising my doctor she would see positive changes in me on my next visit, I would do the same thing. I would go through the drive thru at McDonald's and order 2 Quarter Pounders with cheese and the largest order of fries they made.

Rice cakes are the invention of Betty Crocker's evil twin.

Some people have a fear of clowns. Not me. How could I with Ronald McDonald being such a big part of my life? And with Ronald as my friend, his friend, the Hamburglar also became a close friend of mine.

Speaking of the Hamburglar, little did I know how much was being stolen from me by carrying around over 125 pounds of extra weight.

14 SANTA AND SATAN

Andy Williams reminds us every year in December that "It's the most wonderful time of the year." It should be, and for a lot of people, it is. But for many years, it wasn't for me. Christmas. I was with Scrooge on this one. Bah Humbug!

For the most part, as a kid I wasn't overweight. I may have been a little husky every once in a while. But on average, I was average size.

When I was in 1st grade, I went through a few months of being on the pudgy side. I'll never forget it. Our class was doing a musical to put on for our families. We were doing "Frosty the Snowman." Guess who was asked to play Frosty?

When people say they see my weight loss in my face, I want to know: how big was my face? Was I the Elephant man?

When we were putting on our costumes, I will never forget how the teacher told me that there wasn't much of a need for any extra filling in my costume.

Fast forward about 48 years.

A friend of a friend asks if I

would be willing to help his neighborhood community with their annual children's Christmas party. I was very happy to help. I was thinking I was being asked to donate toys, or help wrap gifts, or supply food. None of that was what they needed from me. This guy asked if I would be their Santa Claus. I know he didn't ask because I could Ho Ho Ho. I was being asked because I was fat, fat, fat.

I was so backed up last week that I was actually hoping somebody would beat the crap out of me.

But that wasn't the worst of it.

I actually had a good time. I had never been a Santa before and I was happy to make a bunch of children happy.

When I was making my exit, I was asked, "Can we count on you being Santa next year?" That sounds innocent enough. But to me, I heard, "Since it's obvious to everyone that you aren't going to be losing weight any time soon, can you roll on down from the North Pole and lend us a hand?"

They tell you to wear black to look thin. Has anybody ever been to Sea World? Have you seen Shamu? He's mostly black.

And then there's the whole Christmas gift thing. People who had no idea of what my size was would buy me clothes. For the record, I haven't been a 2X since the early 1980's. When people bought me a 2X shirt, what were they thinking? What was I to with my other arm?

The only redeeming factor I could find in Christmas was in the cold weather. As long as it was cold and people were bundled up in sweaters and coats, I felt like I wasn't quite as big.

My doctor wants me to step up my exercising... add some jogging. She recommended an APP called "5K the Easy Way." I asked her if she knew of an APP called "Jogging a Lap by Taking a Nap."

Sorry Andy Williams. It wasn't the most wonderful time of the year for me.

And New Years Day, with all those resolutions, wasn't much better.

15 STICKS AND STONES

"Sticks and stones, may break my bones, but words will never harm me."

Words are powerful… sometimes.

When I was overweight, I let some words do a lot of damage to me. I let names that I was called anger me. I allowed things that people said to me dictate how I felt about myself. I permitted my mind to imagine what people were saying or thinking about me.

> *I saw a bunch of guys at the gym the other day that had 6 pack abs, were chiseled, and buff.   It really encouraged me... to quit.*

I let words keep me inside a lot. I would always tell people that I was more of an "inside person." Actually, it was just safer for me to not mingle with people unless it was absolutely necessary.

Words did harm me.

But there were things that people said that I did not allow to affect me like I should have.

When the doctor said I was "pre-

Diabetic," that should have affected me. It didn't.

When the doctor said I was "Diabetic," that should have really impacted me. It didn't for very long.

> *I was so big my wife feared me rolling on top of her and killing her. I told her "Honey, I may crush your body, but I'll never break your heart."*

When the speaker at the pastors conference talked about preachers who are overweight, I should have let that affect me. He said, "When you are overweight, you are just standing in front of your congregation telling everyone that you have no self control." I should have let that sink in. I didn't. I just got mad.

One day Jim, one of my minister friends that travels all over the world, was in town. We arranged to have breakfast together. The meal was wonderful. It was really nice catching up on all that he and his wife had experienced since I had seen him.

Hunger cues are things that make you want to eat. Going to the movies makes you want to eat popcorn. Baseball makes you want to eat hotdogs. What makes me want to eat is... just waking up.

At the close of the meal, Jim said, "John, there's something I need to tell you." He said, "You really need to get your weight under control.

I'm telling you this as a brother and a friend." He went on to say, "If you keep on going down this road, you are going to get so big and so sick that you're going to end up in a wheelchair. And, you are going to weigh so much that your poor little wife isn't going to even be able to push you."

I was offended. I said, "Jim, those are hurtful words. You don't know how strong my wife is!" Okay... that's not exactly what I said.

If you ask me to pray for you to lose weight, tell me how much you want to lose. Why? I need to know how to pray to: Jesus Christ or Jenny Craig.

What I said was nothing. This came out of the blue. I wasn't expecting this. After eating a blueberry muffin, drinking orange juice, and enjoying a couple of cups of coffee, this was the last thing I thought I'd have to deal with.

Always cut your donuts in half, that way you aren't really eating donuts. You're eating "C" food.

I thanked him for his concern and made up something about asking him to pray for me and that I would start working on losing weight. I didn't mean a word of it. I was upset.

I didn't say a word to Jim for over three years. I didn't have anything to say. And I certainly didn't need another sermon.

But Jim was absolutely right.

If things didn't turn around, I most definitely would be fulfilling his prophecy.

Ever since that meeting, blueberry muffins just don't taste the same. Now don't think I gave them up, because I most certainly didn't. It wasn't the muffin that offended me.

16 WALLET AND WEIGHT

I hated going to the doctor. It seemed that a doctor visit always meant another pill.

Whenever the physician's assistant would check my vitals, I would always do the same thing. I would take everything out of my pockets, wallet, keys, coins, everything, including my handkerchief and comb. It's something about a comb that can make the scales give you a bad number. As I unloaded my pockets, I would tell the PA, "I need to make sure the scales show all my hard work."

The day that my doctor told me that I was a Diabetic, I can't say that I was surprised. I didn't do anything to prevent it. But that day I was determined to reverse that diagnosis.

They say you learn more from your mistakes than your successes. If that's true, I must be a freakin' genius.

I went home, changed clothes, and walked the neighborhood park for 45 minutes. I did the same thing the next day and the next. I did this, without missing a day for 6 months.

I dropped about 40 pounds.

Then like everything else positive that I had ever done for my body, I quit. I don't even know why. I just quit.

> I was told to "Vote my conscience." So... I'm voting for pizza and his running mate, lemon pepper chicken wings.

The weight all came back and more. It was at this time that I became a part of the 300 Club. I was now weighing over 300 pounds.

I couldn't believe that I had let myself reach this point.

Or maybe I do believe it.

I didn't do anything to curtail my

bad eating habits.

Whenever my wife and I would pick up food at a drive thru (and this was always at my suggestion, or rather, arm twisting, because my wife knew better), I would, at a minimum, order two burgers and the largest order of fries the establishment had to offer. My wife would want a "small" whatever it was we were going to eat. But I would order her a large because I wanted to make sure she had leftovers that I would be consuming.

> *Application: What have you done in your life that you are most proud of? Me: Not dying.*

My wife was never happy with my

dietary choices. She tried to convince me to change my ways, but I didn't.

For a stress test, you no longer have to get on a treadmill. Now you just go to the billing department.

I just loved food. It didn't even have to be all that good as long as there was lots of it.

I didn't smoke, drink, or do drugs. I just ate too much.

Some people say things like: "I don't know how it happened. I just woke up one day overweight." Well, I know how my obesity happened. I did it to myself. I'm not blaming anyone. It was all me.

If things were going to change, it

Laughing My Butt Off

was going to take a miracle.

17 KIDDING AND KIDNEY STONES

One day as my doctor was making her notes on my condition, I saw her write something that was quite alarming: "morbid obesity."

I asked her what that meant. She said it meant that my weight was actually life threatening.

I asked what weight I needed to be to change that diagnosis. She said, "Below 250."

I was 74 pounds away.

I thought, "That's impossible."

I don't know where cheesecake fits into this new diet... but I'm sure I can squeeze it in.

Why kid myself into thinking I could get there?

I didn't do anything for a while to try to lose my title of being morbidly obese.

And then the kidney stones began.

One night I couldn't sleep. I tossed and turned and couldn't find a comfortable position to get my body in. My lower back was killing me. Tylenol, no matter how many I took, did nothing to alleviate the pain.

> *Go to my doctor. He gives a 25% discount on the treatment of any disease caught while sitting in his waiting room.*

When the pain got unbearable, I drove myself to the closest emergency room. They immediately diagnosed me as having kidney stones. I was given a few pain killers, Flowmax, and told to make an appointment with a urologist.

By the time I saw the urologist, I had already passed the stones. He told me I needed to lose weight, change my diet, or this would not be an isolated episode.

When I was out of the woods and the pain was gone, I was back to my old ways.

Until the kidney stones returned.

My urologist sent me to the hospital where I underwent Shock Wave Lithotripsy. This is a procedure where the stones are broken apart so they will pass.

> *My friend found out the hard way that "to be euthanized" does not mean "to be made to look younger."*

The procedure was a success. The stones that were creating the blockage were dissolved. However, my urologist told me that there were new stones forming and that I really needed to change my ways.

I changed immediately. After the procedure, I went to a different restaurant for breakfast.

The motivational speaker told me to "always look up." Now I'm looking up "chiropractor" in the Yellow Pages.

Once the pain was gone, so was any thought of a change in my life.

And then the stones came back again.

My urologist told me that he could not perform the Lithotripsy procedure again because of my size. He said that I was too big and the table would collapse.

Thankfully, those stones passed on their own after a couple of days.

My urologist sent me to see a kidney specialist. This new doctor told me that if I would do exactly what he told me that I would never have a kidney stone attack again. He told me to avoid certain foods and take a certain prescription drug.

Believe it or not, I did what he told me and he was right. It's been over five years since I have had a kidney stone.

My weight loss has had a world-wide impact. 14 countries have now been removed from the "Starving to Death Because There's No Food" list.

On top of this, I lost some weight. I dropped about 60 pounds.

But after months of pain-free living, I went back to my old ways and gained about 55 of those 60 lost pounds.

I didn't think I could feel any worse about myself. Then the dentist informed me that I was born without wisdom teeth.

I was on a roller coaster ride that seemed to never end.

18 LOSING AND LAPSING

I finally cancelled my membership to the 300 Club.

My therapist recommended "self talk." I've gotten so good at it that now I have multiple personality disorder.

I had made it to the 290's and I had my next visit to the doctor. She was happy to see the scale going in the right direction. I asked her what

I had asked months before, "At what point do I get out of the morbid obesity category?" She said, "When you get below 250."

> *With my multiple personality disorder, no wonder I'm overweight. 16 people are living in here.*

So I made 249 a goal.

I even attached a reward to my goal. I told myself that I was going to be a new person and wanted the look to match. I set a goal to shave off my moustache. I had had it for over 20 years. But I decided it would go when the extra weight left.

For the next few months, I did pretty good. I tried cutting down on what I was eating and I started walking. I tried to walk at least 30 minutes 5 times a week but usually I only got about 3 walks in. But I was still making progress.

It took about nine months for me to hit 249. I was very proud of myself. I felt like I could lose a lot more.

The moustache came off. The new look seemed to shave about 10 years off my age, too. This helped me stay motivated.

My therapist is outrageous. She's giving a bill to each of my personalities.

I kept with my new regimen of eating less and walking a few times a week.

I made it to 244.

And then Winter made her annual appearance.

The excuses began.

> *My therapist is firing me as a patient. But... she says my multiple personalities can keep continuing seeing her.*

It's too cold.

The wind is blowing too hard.

It's too hard to walk wearing a coat.

I forgot my knit cap.

One excuse after another.

So basically, I went the entire three months of Winter doing very little. But I did eat… too much.

Sadly, I gained 40 or so pounds and regained my title of "morbidly obese."

The church is building a New Life Center. It's really more of an "after life" center. Actually, it's a mausoleum.

Over the years through my weight struggle, people would ask me if I considered getting a lapband or having gastric bypass surgery. I never gave those procedures much of a thought. I always felt like I had what it took to get the weight off if I'd just stick with it.

John W. Turner

But I didn't have what it took.

Something was missing and I had no clue as to what it was.

19 LEARNING AND LIVING

A couple more years had gone by without any real progress with my weight. During this time, my doctor went into private practice and I got a new doctor.

Therapists have come up with a way to help people with low self esteem. They have created a new level called "lower self esteem."

Nothing changed.

In January of 2016, I had my next doctor's appointment. Like usual, I dreaded the visit. It would be more bad news, probably the addition of another pill, and more of me feeling bad about myself.

But, believe it or not, this time was different.

NASA can send a rover to Mars, 249 million miles away, examine a dirt speck in great detail, send the results to Houston, all in less than a second. So why can't my urologist examine my prostate without sticking his finger in my behind?

When the doctor entered the room, she asked, "How's it going?"

I said, "Not too good. I fell off the wagon over the holidays." Truthfully, I didn't just fall off the wagon, I fell off, and then I ate the wagon.

I weighed 274 pounds.

Then I added, "I sure hope you have a magic bullet."

It's pretty bad when the best thing that happens in your day is saving 15% or more on your car insurance.

My doctor said, "I don't have a magic bullet, but I do know what will help you. It's helped a lot of my patients and I've seen a lot of success stories."

What began in the next 5 minutes

in her office, was what I had been missing the last 30 years.

Education.

Nothing had been working to help me get healthy because there were some things I didn't know.

It has been said that "Inspiration without education leads only to frustration."

I had heard that quote in a sermon. It made sense the way the preacher applied it. But I never thought about it in relationship to my fitness and wellbeing.

> *Do laps around the buffet tables at Golden Corral count as exercise?*

The things I was about to learn were not mind-blowing. It was as if I already knew them, but needed a reminder.

The information that I gathered and the application of it have completely turned my life around.

In the next chapter, I will share with you what I learned to do that helped me lose 125 pounds. These are things that almost anyone can do and none of them involve a surgeon's knife or a weird shake to drink.

20 SIXTY THINGS I DID TO LOSE OVER 125 POUNDS

1. I decided to get healthy. No one else convinced me, forced me, or guilted me. I didn't start getting healthy because of my wife, my doctor, concerned friends, or anyone else. This was a decision I made in my time.

2. I followed good advice. My doctor encouraged me to learn about diabetes, nutrition, exercise,

and my body. The educational piece was what was missing in my life all those years. Knowing was the key to going in the right direction.

3. I started. I love the story of the five frogs that sat on a log. One decided to leap off. How many frogs were left on the log? Five? No. Four. Because making a decision doesn't change anything. Doing changes things. So I started.

4. I food journaled. I wrote down everything I consumed. Food, beverages, snacks, etc.

5. I wrote down the calories of everything I consumed.

6. I found out how many fat grams per day I was allowed for my

weight.   (You can research this online.)

7. I wrote down the fat grams of everything I ate or drank.

8. I faced the truth that I was eating way more fat than I should have been eating.

9. I brainstormed ways I could cut the fat.

10. I eliminated some items in my diet that were high in fat.

11. I limited the portion size of some of the items in my diet to cut fat grams.

12. I found "fat free" or "low fat" alternatives to what I was eating. I

discovered there were fat free cheeses, a fat free mayonnaise, a fat free dry cream for coffee, fat free salad dressings, etc.

13. I replaced some fat high foods with foods with less fat content. Instead of half of a jar of dry roasted peanuts, I ate a cucumber with Fat Free Dressing.

14. I brought my fat intake within the designated limits.

15. I didn't skip meals. I used to think that skipping a meal would be helpful. It wasn't. It just made me hungrier when I did eat and then I would eat more.

16. I worked on avoiding late night eating as much as possible.

17. I started exercising seriously. My exercise of choice is walking. When I started, I could only walk a few blocks, but I did it.

18. I removed food temptations from the house. Thankfully, my wife was completely on board with this new lifestyle, so we were both in agreement to get rid of foods that were not healthy for us.

19. I wrote a health conscious shopping list.

20. I made sure there were healthy foods to eat in the house.

21. When I would eat out, I would look for the healthy alternatives on the menu.

22. If I had advanced warning of where I would be eating out, I would look up that restaurant's menu online before going and make decisions before I arrived.

23. I had to prepare myself mentally for the comments and questions around the table. "Are you sure you want just a salad?" "One pizza won't hurt you." "Are you sure you don't want enchiladas?"

24. I would take a healthy lunch to work.

25. If I was going to be travelling at meal time, I would bring my lunch, something I could keep iced down in the car.

26. I increased my walking. I went from a few blocks to a mile. I went from one mile to 1½ miles... then to 2 miles, then 3, etc.

27. I mixed up my walking by walking in different places.

28. I found ways to make walking fun. I always have my cell phone with me and I really enjoy looking for things to photograph. I love taking selfies of my fitness journey.

29. I sometimes listen to podcasts on my walk. Walking time can also be learning time.

30. As I lost weight, I would go on an occasional hike on a nature trail.

31. I challenged myself. Can I walk 5 miles? 8 miles? 10 miles?

32. I set walking goals. My next goal is to walk a half marathon.

33. I kept an umbrella nearby. As soon as I decided to start walking, it rained. When it stopped raining, it was cold. When it began to warm up, it was too hot. So many excuses kept me from exercising. I began to prepare so the excuses could be removed. I kept an umbrella handy in case it was raining. I decided I would rather be a little wet than a whole lot dead. When it was hot, I'd wear a tank top and shorts. I am not yet to the point where I am ready to go shirtless. When it was cold, I'd wear a sweater, warm-ups, or a coat.

34. When my schedule got changed, I didn't remove exercise. There were specific times I would go out for my walk. Whenever there was a schedule conflict, in the beginning of this journey, exercise got eliminated. I learned to readjust my schedule. Most of my exercise regimen is walking outside. It didn't take me long to realize that no matter how full my day was, outside never closes.

35. I discovered that if exercise is first on my list, even if extremely early in the morning, it will always get done.

36. I weighed every day. Some suggest that you only weigh once a week. Not me. I weigh every day. When I get up in the morning, after

I go to the bathroom, the next thing I do is weigh myself. I do this to encourage myself if there is weight loss. If I haven't lost, knowing my weight is a motivator throughout the day. I record my weight daily to keep track of the progress.

37. I did not have cheat days. When people start new fitness and health plans, it seems that everyone feels like you need cheat days. I have friends that even have cheat weeks. I don't cheat on my diet and fitness. I know that bending my new lifestyle would be the beginning of ending my new lifestyle. You may be strong enough to bounce back. I know I'm not. I have an occasional "treat." Yesterday, I was at my sister-in-laws birthday party. I ate a very slender slice of cake. No

ice cream. No punch. This was a treat. And then later in the day during my dinner, I eliminated my dessert.

38. I learned that a taste was all I needed. On my wedding anniversary, I took my wife out to eat. We went to one of our favorite Mexican food restaurants. We selected a reasonably healthy plate. And then came the tortillas. The tortillas at this restaurant are, as they say, "to die for." In the past, I would usually eat 5 or 6 of them covered with butter. On this particular evening, I surprised myself. My wife and I split one tortilla. We learned that a taste was just enough. It satisfied that desire to have tortillas.

39.   I redefined "extra time" as "exercise time."   If a small window of time opened up in my schedule, I would take advantage of it by going for a walk.

40. I gave myself a lot of "whys." The reasons I have for this new lifestyle keep me going.   A few of my reasons are: I wanted to feel better. I wanted to be able to shop at regular stores for clothes. I wanted to get off my prescription drugs.   I wanted to be alive and active to enjoy my granddaughter.

41. I took baby steps.   It may sound like I made a lot of huge changes, but they were all small ones in the beginning.

42.   I found a plan that works for

me. I don't really like to call it a plan. "Plan" sounds a lot like "diet." I just found a healthy way of living that I could live with. You will have to find what works for you. One size does not fit all.

43. I became accountable to myself. That's what my food journal is all about. Knowing that I will be writing down everything I eat and facing those facts on paper, helps me.

44. I also became accountable to someone else. When I began to make these changes, I made myself accountable to someone else. This was my choice. Knowing I would be sharing results, helped me. It helps to receive the encouragement. I continue to do this.

45. I got a fitness partner. She happens to be my wife. We do this together.

46. I filled my life with positive motivation. I read books written by runners. One of my favorites is Dean Karnazes, ultra-marathon runner.

47. I pushed myself. I always hit invisible walls when I walk. I hit one during the first 5 minutes. That wall tells me "Stop, turn around, you're too busy." I have to push through to get started. Then about one third of the way through I hit another wall. That wall tells me "You've done enough, you're tired, you hurt." But, again. I push through.

48. I kept a chart of my progress on the wall. As I am writing this, I was able to record that fact that I have officially unjoined The Two Hundred Club. I saw the number "199" on the scale for the first time since the early 1980's. My chart encourages me on this journey.

49. I set goals for myself. Some of my goals involved my weight and others involved my walking.

50. I ate out less. I used to eat out for most of my meals. This new lifestyle has me in the kitchen cooking more and loving it. It has also greatly benefited our finances.

51. I avoided the meal before the meal. On those rare occasions that I would eat out, I kept myself from

the tortilla chips, or bread, or whatever the restaurant would give me before my plate ever arrived on the table.

52.   I believed that I could accomplish weight loss without pills, surgeries, procedures, or some expensive program. I am not critical of those who may need some form of weight loss surgery. You know your situation. I am speaking about those who can make the changes without a procedure.

53. I received and welcomed compliments. I posted a lot of selfies as I started out on this journey.   Lots   of   folks complimented my progress. I was greatly benefited by knowing that so many people cared about my health.

54. I did not receive into my spirit words that did not help me. People who meant well would tell me things like: "You look good the way you are." "Don't change." "It's good to have a little meat on your bones." "You've lost too much weight. Are you sick?" I couldn't stop people from saying those things, but I did not have to make them a part of my life.

55. I quit playing the blame game. I used to blame my parents for the "fat" gene. I blamed work for a bad schedule. I blamed my friends and their peer pressure to make me eat wrong. I blamed church for always having food at every gathering. But the truth is, I was to blame. No one force fed me. It was all me.

56. I got rid of my big clothes. I made sure I didn't have a backup plan in case I gained weight. I have only one pair of my size 50 pants just to show people where I used to be.

57. I didn't wait for everyone else to get on the band wagon. Thankfully, my wife is on the same page with me. But I didn't wait for my entire family or all of my coworkers to decide to get healthy. I am a self starter. I'm self motivated. And this worked to my advantage in this new healthy lifestyle.

58. I wanted to help others. For the last 32 years, I have been a pastor. I have spent almost my entire life helping people. Now, I

want to help people lose weight.

59. I wanted to write this book. Several years ago, I heard a motivational speaker talk about going to his publisher with his next book idea. He said he was going to write a book about how he lost 60 pounds. He said the book would be finished in 6 months. At the time, he had not lost the 60 pounds. But the publisher's deadline was his motivator. In 6 months, the book was finished and the weight was off. I wanted to do that. I have had this book in my mind for several years. When I got serious about my weight loss, I allowed the completion of this book to be one of my goals, as well.

60. I did it. It wasn't thinking,

wishing, hoping, praying, believing, or wanting. It was all about doing. And it still is. One of the most important phrases in the Bible is: "faith without works is dead." It took work to get to where I am today. Hard work? Yes. But rewarding. Worth it? Absolutely. Impossible work? No. It's possible. I am living proof. If I can do it, you can do it.

21 ABC'S AND 1,2,3'S

I love simplicity.

If you were to ask me to simplify my new healthy lifestyle into 3 points, I could.

> *Things could be worse. You could be that guy who lost his glass eye in the produce section of the grocery store.*

First, letter "a" stands for Accountability. My whole new way of living is about staying accountable to myself. I do this with my daily food journal, wall chart record of my weight, and with my printed sheets of my goals. I also stay accountable to a few people that I have chosen to be my fellow partners on this journey. All I do is let them know about my progress on a regular basis. As simple as that is, it is huge in my life.

The first step of the journey is not the hardest. The first step off a skyscraper is.

Second, letter "b" stands for Body Moving. For me, this is about walking. It is about getting my body into some kind of exercise for at least 30 minutes, 5 times a week.

Third, letter "c" stands for Cut Fat. That's the major change in my eating. I have opted for a low fat lifestyle. It seems that just removing the large amount of fat that I was consuming, has considerably cut my weight.

22 TRUNKS AND TERROR

Remember my graduation robe horror story? It all came back to haunt me the other day.

I had not seen my brother Bill for months and decided to make a visit out to his house and spend the day with him. It was great. We went for a hike together and then spent a few hours with two of his grandsons, my grand-nephews.

In the middle of the afternoon, my brother suggested we all go swimming at the pool in his subdivision. I let him know that I didn't bring any swimming trunks. He said, "Don't worry. I have an extra pair."

The commercial on TV says: Inside every overweight person is a skinny person trying to get out. That explains the extra 100 pounds.

As he went to go get the trunks, I thought about Robert, the graduation coordinator, when he handed me that robe that was way too small. I could hear his voice again saying, "Lots of people wear them unzipped."

My brother has always been fit

and trim, if you ask me. In my mind, I could see him bringing me some trunks that were way too small. I could see myself not fitting into them. And, I could hear him saying, "Lots of people wear them unzipped."

Argghhhhhh!!!!

> *I got good news from my therapist. I don't have low self esteem. I actually am a loser.*

But that's not what happened.

My brother handed me the trunks. I thought for sure they were too small. But they weren't. I didn't have to wear them unzipped to the pool.

That day, it hit me: I really have changed. I am living a new lifestyle.

I can fit into other people's clothes without having to wear them unzipped.

You know you're getting old when people buy you clothes for your birthday... especially when they buy you a shroud.

And on that note, I will zip up my mouth, that is guiding my typing hands, and end this book.

23 CONCLUSION

As this book goes to press, I weigh 198 pounds. This is 126 pounds less than my highest recorded weight at the doctor's office. I am sure that I was well over 350 pounds at my heaviest. My A1C has dropped from a 6.2 to a 5.9. I no longer have high blood pressure. My BMI has gone from

39.31 to 32.28. I have gone from taking 6 prescription drugs to taking ½ of one pill a day.

I no longer wear a size 50 pants. I wear a size 38. I wear a large or XL shirt and not a 4X.

I feel better than I have ever felt in my life.

I lost the weight that was holding me back from living my life. It was done without pills, surgery, or alfalfa sprouts.

If I can do it, you can do it.

You can lose the weight and at the very same time, laugh your butt off.

ABOUT THE AUTHOR

John W. Turner is a comedian, pastor, author, poet, spiritual advisor, husband, stepfather, grandfather, uncle, friend, etc. But here's what you really want to know since you have picked up this book: John is just a normal person like you. He has struggled with his weight for most of his adult life. He tried a lot of things to lose the weight and got really fed up being on the weight rollercoaster.

Thanks to what you will read in this book, John has his weight under control.

John W. Turner